Sex Without Bonds:

Navigating Physical Intimacy Without Emotional Ties

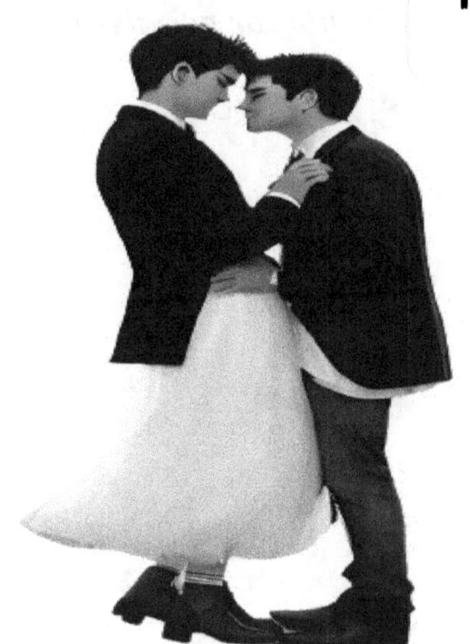

Ann R. Disanto

TABLE OF CONTENTS

Introduction

In a world increasingly__ fueled by instant connections and spontaneous encounters, our perceptions of intimacy have undergone a radical transformation. The very fabric of human relationships is being rewoven with threads of modern desires, technology's__ influence, and the persistent quest for emotional equilibrium. ENTER THE REALM Of "Sex Without Bonds: Navigating Physical Intimacy Without Emotional Ties".

Many have asked, is it truly possible to separate the passionate whirlwind of physical __intimacy from the deep, often turbulent waters of emotional attachment? This isn't just a question of casual liaisons, but a deeper__ exploration into the human psyche, our needs, and our boundaries.

With societal__ norms shifting, many find solace in the freedom of emotional independence. For some, casual relationships offer an avenue to explore without the weight of commitment, while for others, they are a means of self-discovery, a journey devoid of traditional __expectations. But how does one traverse this path without getting ensnared in the emotional undercurrents?

This book seeks to demystify the labyrinth of human connections. It's an invitation to embark on an__ enlightening journey – to understand the science of attachment, to embrace the art of clear _communication, and to safeguard one's emotional and physical well-being.

Whether you're a curious soul, a skeptic, or someone who has __experienced the complexities of emotion-free intimacy, there's something in these pages for you. Prepare to challenge your preconceptions, equip yourself with valuable __insights, and perhaps even redefine your understanding of modern relationships.

Welcome to a discourse that promises to be as__ intriguing as it is enlightening. Dive in, and let's navigate the intricate dance of physical__ intimacy without the confines of emotional bonds.

Part I: Understanding Emotional Bonds

Emotional bonds, often seen as the invisible__ threads connecting us to others, are fundamental to human relationships. Their role in our lives is multi-dimensional:

1. **Nature of Emotional Bonds:** At the core, emotional__ bonds are a blend of affection, trust, and dependency. They are the feelings that make us want to be closer to someone, to__ seek their company, and to care for their well-being.

2. **Origins:** Emotional__ connections often find their roots in early childhood. BONDS FORMED with PRIMARY CAREGIVERS lay the groundwork for FUTURE__ RELATIONSHIPS. The trust, security, or lack thereof, experienced during these early years can greatly influence our later attachments.

3. **Attachment Styles:** Researchers have identified several attachment styles - Secure, Anxious, Avoidant, and Disorganized. Each__ style affects how we perceive and engage in relationships. Recognizing one's style can be crucial in understanding our __reactions and behaviors in intimate situations.

4. **Emotional Bonds vs. Physical Intimacy:** It's a misconception that physical intimacy always fosters deep emotional ties. While physical__ closeness can enhance bonds, it doesn't inherently create them. Many factors, including__ communication, shared experiences, and mutual respect, play a role in deepening emotional connections.

5. **The Impact of Culture and Society:** Cultural norms, societal expectations, and personal__ experiences shape our understanding of emotional bonds. In some cultures, deep emotional connections are expected to precede physical__ intimacy, while in others, casual relationships without profound emotional ties are common and acceptable.

6. **Benefits and Challenges:** Emotional bonds are double-edged. On one hand, they can offer__ support, security, and deep understanding. On the other hand, when these bonds are unhealthy or one-sided, they can lead to emotional_ turmoil, dependency, or even heartbreak.

In this section, we'll delve deep into the intricate__ world of emotional bonds, examining their origins, their nature, and their impact on our lives. By understanding these__ ties, we are better equipped to navigate relationships that prioritize physical intimacy without the intertwined emotions.

Part II: The Benefits of Keeping Distance

Maintaining a certain distance in relationships, especially when emphasizing physical__ intimacy over emotional attachment, offers numerous advantages:

1. **Emotional Autonomy:** Without deep emotional ties, individuals can retain their emotional__ independence, making decisions without the weight of another's feelings influencing them.

2. **Flexibility:** Distance can provide the flexibility to explore different_ facets of oneself and engage in multiple relationships, learning from varied experiences without the complexities of deep emotional __entanglements.

3. **Avoiding Emotional Drain:** Relationships, especially those with emotional_ depth, can sometimes lead to__ exhaustion. Keeping distance

can help individuals sidestep the potential emotional drain that deeper_ connections might bring.

4. **Clarity in Intentions:** When both parties understand and respect the boundaries, there's less_ room for misunderstanding. The focus remains on mutual_ enjoyment without the expectations of traditional commitment.

5. **Personal Growth:** Without the need to constantly cater to a partner's_ emotional needs, individuals can focus more on personal__ growth, self-discovery, and pursuing individual passions.

6. **Safety Net Against Heartbreak:** While no strategy is foolproof against emotional hurt, maintaining__ distance can act as a buffer. The emotional stakes are different, often leading to less profound_ pain in case of a breakup.

7. **Simplified Complications:** With fewer emotional ties, the complexities often associated with__ jealousy, possessiveness, and high expectations can be minimized, leading to simpler, more straightforward_ interactions.

In this section, we emphasize the value of maintaining__ distance in certain relationships, exploring the manifold benefits it can bring to personal well-being, growth, and the overall dynamics of casual_ connections.

Part III: Practical Steps to Navigating Sex Without Bonds

Embarking on a journey of physical intimacy without deep__ emotional ties requires clarity, communication, and self-awareness. Here are concrete steps to ensure a healthy_ experience:

1. **Open Communication:** Begin every relationship with transparent conversations about intentions. Make sure both __parties are on the same page regarding expectations.

2. **Set Clear Boundaries:** Determine what behaviors are __acceptable and what aren't. This could range from frequency of meetups to topics of conversation post-intimacy.

3. **Regular Check-ins:** Periodically discuss feelings and ensure that the relationship hasn't inadvertently __shifted into emotional territory.

4. **Limit Shared Personal Details:** While openness is vital, be cautious about sharing deeply personal__ stories or details that may foster unintended emotional connections.

5. **Prioritize Safety:** Always practice safe sex. This includes regular health check-ups and open__ discussions about sexual health.

6. **Avoid Traditional Dating Settings:** To prevent sending mixed signals, consider avoiding __romantic dinner dates or meeting family and friends. Opt for neutral settings instead.

7. **Stay Informed:** Educate yourself on the emotional and psychological_ implications of casual__ relationships to navigate potential pitfalls.

8. **Emotional Preparedness:** Be ready for unexpected emotions. It's natural to feel attachment even with__ precautions. Have strategies in place to cope and reassess.

9. **Listen to Your Gut:** If something feels off or you suspect deeper__ feelings are forming, it might be time to step back and evaluate.

10. **Have an Exit Strategy:** Every relationship has an endpoint. Understand when it's time to move on and have a respectful way to __communicate this.

In this section, we offer a roadmap to approach physical__ intimacy without emotional ties. It's about ensuring mutual respect, understanding, and prioritizing one's well-being.

Part IV: The Role of Self-awareness and Mindfulness

Harnessing self-awareness and mindfulness is paramount in navigating relationships without deep _emotional ties. HERE'S HOW THEY PLAY A CRITICAL ROLE:

1. **Recognizing Motivations:** Being self-aware helps you understand why you're seeking casual __connections. Are they for exploration, healing from past relationships, or just momentary pleasure?

2. **Staying Present:** Mindfulness allows you to be present during intimate moments, making them more__ genuine and ensuring you don't inadvertently delve into emotional_ territories.

3. **Emotional Regulation:** Practicing mindfulness helps regulate__ emotions, ensuring that feelings don't escalate unchecked.

4. **Identifying Triggers:** Self-awareness will help you pinpoint triggers that might lead to unwanted emotional __attachments, enabling you to address them proactively.

5. **Self-compassion:** It's vital to approach oneself with kindness, especially when navigating complex__ relationships. Mindfulness fosters a non-judgmental perspective towards oneself.

6. **Enhanced Communication:** Being in tune with one's feelings can lead to clearer, more transparent__ conversations with partners.

7. **Boundaries Check:** Regularly practicing self-awareness helps in ensuring that set boundaries are not being_ crossed, allowing for adjustments as needed.

8. **Mindful Intimacy:** Being mindful during physical__ encounters can enhance the experience, making it richer and more fulfilling without delving into emotional depth.

9. **Clarity in Choices:** With heightened self-awareness, decisions are made more consciously, ensuring that they align with one's true__ desires and intentions.

In this section, we emphasize the importance of turning__ inward, understanding oneself, and leveraging mindfulness as a tool to navigate the intricacies of relationships without bonds.

Part V: Perspectives from Different Genders and Orientations

Sexual__ experiences without emotional ties can be perceived and navigated differently across genders and orientations. Here's a breakdown:

1. **Male Perspective:** Often societal norms may pressure men to disconnect_ emotion from sex. Understanding these influences and stereotypes can provide clarity on genuine personal __feelings versus conditioned responses.

2. **Female Perspective:** Women, traditionally seen as the more emotionally-inclined gender, may grapple with different__ expectations and pressures. Exploring this can help in understanding the nuances of their experiences in casual_ relationships.

3. **LGBTQ+ Community:** The spectrum of experiences in the LGBTQ+ community is vast. Perspectives here might differ based on societal__

acceptance, personal struggles, and the fluidity of relationships.

4. **Non-Binary & Genderqueer:** People who don't identify strictly as male or female may have unique__ experiences and challenges in separating emotion from intimacy, influenced by their personal journey and societal responses.

5. **Cultural Influences:** Different cultures have distinct views on gender__ roles, sexual freedom, and emotional expression, all of which can influence perspectives on sex without_ bonds.

6. **Emotional Conditioning:** It's important to address how emotional responses to physical__ intimacy can be conditioned differently based on one's gender or orientation, resulting from societal expectations or personal_ experiences.

7. **Breaking Stereotypes:** An exploration of how different genders and orientations are challenging traditional_ views on casual relationships and forging their own paths.

In this section, we delve into the diverse experiences of different _genders and orientations, understanding how each navigates the terrain of sex without deep emotional _connections.

Part VI: Health and Safety in Casual Relationships

Navigating casual__ relationships requires a keen emphasis on health and safety to ensure positive experiences for all involved:

1. **Sexual Health:** Prioritize regular testing and safe sex practices. Openly discuss sexual health __histories with partners.

2. **Emotional Well-being:** Recognize the importance of emotional__ safety. Ensure that casual relationships don't negatively impact mental health.

3. **Consent:** An absolute cornerstone. Every intimate act should be consensual, with clear__ communication about boundaries and comfort levels.

4. **Avoid Substance Reliance:** Be cautious about relying on alcohol or drugs during encounters, as they can cloud _judgment and compromise_ safety.

5. **Recognizing Red_ Flags:** Stay alert to signs of possessiveness, disrespect, or any form of emotional or physical_ abuse.

6. **Privacy:** Protect your personal information. Be cautious about sharing details that could__ compromise your privacy or safety.

7. **Safe Meeting Practices:** Always meet in public__ places when getting to know someone. Inform a trusted_ person about your whereabouts.

8. **Trust Your Instincts:** If something feels off, it probably is. Listen to your gut feelings about_ situations or individuals.

9. **Aftercare:** Especially if engaging in intense physical__ encounters, ensure that there's a level of aftercare to address physical and emotional well-being.

10. **Exit Strategies:** Have a plan in place for ending the relationship or encounter safely if it no longer_ aligns with your comfort or desires.

In this section, we underscore the critical aspects of maintaining one's_ health and safety while_ exploring casual relationships, ensuring that every interaction is respectful, consensual, and positive.

Conclusion

In the intricate dance of human connections, the line between physical intimacy and emotional_ ties often blurs. As we've journeyed through the multifaceted_ world of "Sex Without Bonds," we've unraveled the complexities of relationships that prioritize the physical over the emotional, while also emphasizing the importance of self-awareness, health, and safety.

Our modern age, with its evolving societal norms and varied individual_ perspectives, offers the opportunity to define relationships on our own terms. While the concept of separating_ sex from deep emotional bonds may be challenging for some, for others, it represents freedom, exploration, and personal_ growth.

What remains paramount, regardless of one's choice, is mutual_ respect, clear communication, and a deep understanding of one's_ desires and boundaries. Every relationship, casual or deep-rooted, should be approached with care, consciousness, and compassion.

As you move forward, may you carry the insights and perspectives_ shared in these pages, ensuring that each connection you forge is genuine, safe, and fulfilling, irrespective of its_ depth or duration.

Thank you for deciding to purchase this book. Your support means a lot to me, and I hope you find it informative and entertaining to read.

If you have the time, I would be grateful if you could leave a review for the book. Your feedback enables me to improve while also providing useful _ information to other potential readers.

Thank you once more for your assistance, and best _ wishes on your journey.